FIVE WEIGHT LOSS SECRETS

A Comprehensive Diet Plan
for Lasting Results

By

Dr. Mike Edwards

Table of contents

Introduction

Welcome to "The Ultimate Guide to Sustainable Weight Loss: A Comprehensive Diet Plan for Lasting Results." This book is designed to help you achieve your weight loss goals through a sustainable and realistic approach to diet and exercise.

Losing weight is a journey that can be both challenging and rewarding. While there are many diets and weight loss plans available, not all of them are sustainable or healthy in the long term. This book is different. We will focus on creating a healthy, balanced diet plan that suits your lifestyle and preferences, and provide you with the tools and strategies you need to stay motivated and on track.

In this book, we will start by exploring the science of weight loss and metabolism. You'll learn how your body gains and loses weight, and how to create a calorie deficit that promotes fat loss. We'll also discuss the importance of setting realistic goals, identifying obstacles and creating a plan to overcome them, and staying motivated and accountable.

Next, we'll dive into the heart of the book: creating your personalized meal plan. We'll help you assess your dietary needs and preferences, design a meal plan that suits your lifestyle, and provide tips for meal prep and dining out.

We'll also discuss the importance of making healthy choices every day, including strategies for managing cravings and emotional eating. We'll talk about the benefits of exercise for weight loss and overall health, and provide tips for staying active and motivated.

Finally, we'll explore common challenges that arise during weight loss, such as plateaus and setbacks, and provide strategies for overcoming them. We'll also talk about how to maintain a healthy weight for life.

By the end of this book, you'll have the knowledge and tools you need to achieve sustainable weight loss and maintain a healthy lifestyle. Let's get started!

Chapter 1: The science of Weight Loss: What You Need to Know

Losing weight can be a challenging process, but understanding the science behind weight loss can make it easier to achieve your goals. In this chapter, we'll explore how your body gains and loses weight, the role of metabolism in weight loss, and the importance of calories and macronutrients.

How Your Body Gains and Loses Weight

When you ingest more calories than you expend, weight increase results. Your body stores excess calories as fat, which can lead to weight gain over time. Conversely, weight loss occurs when you burn more calories than you consume. Your body breaks down fat stores to provide energy, leading to weight loss.

However, weight loss isn't always as simple as "calories in, calories out." Your body is a complex system that is influenced by many factors, including genetics, hormones, and lifestyle factors. That's why it's important to take a comprehensive approach to weight loss, focusing on both diet and exercise.

The Role of Metabolism in Weight Loss

Metabolism refers to the chemical processes in your body that convert food into energy. Your metabolism is influenced by many factors, including age, gender, body composition, and genetics.

The function of metabolism in weight reduction is significant. Your metabolism determines how many calories you burn at rest, also known as your basal metabolic rate (BMR). By increasing your BMR through exercise and building muscle, you can burn more calories throughout the day and promote weight loss.

The Importance of Calories and Macronutrients

Calories are a measure of energy. When it comes to weight loss, it's important to consume fewer calories than you burn. However, not all calories are created equal. The types of food you eat can influence your weight loss journey.

Macronutrients are the three main types of nutrients that provide energy: carbohydrates, protein, and fat. Each macronutrient plays a different role in your body, and the amount you need depends on your individual needs and goals.

Carbohydrates are your body's main source of energy. However, not all carbohydrates are created equal. Complex carbohydrates, such as whole grains, fruits, and vegetables, are more filling and provide more sustained energy than simple carbohydrates, such as sugar and processed foods.

Protein is essential for building and repairing tissue in your body. It's also important for maintaining muscle mass, which can help increase your BMR and promote weight loss.

Fat is important for many bodily functions, including hormone production and nutrient absorption. However, not all fats are created equal. Unsaturated fats, such as those found in nuts, seeds, and fatty fish, are healthier than saturated and trans fats, which can increase your risk of heart disease.

In the next chapter, we'll explore how to use this knowledge to create a personalized meal plan for sustainable weight loss.

Chapter 2: Building a Foundation for Lasting Success

Before diving into a weight loss plan, it's important to build a foundation for lasting success. In this chapter, we'll explore the importance of setting realistic goals, identifying obstacles and creating a plan to overcome them, and staying motivated and accountable.

Setting Realistic Goals

Achieving sustainable weight reduction depends on setting reasonable objectives. Your objectives ought to be time-bound, pertinent, measurable, and precise. Instead of stating that you want to "lose weight," for instance, make your aim to "lose 10 pounds by following a healthy diet plan and exercising three times per week" instead.

Identifying Obstacles and Creating a Plan to Overcome Them

Obstacles can arise during any weight loss journey. It's important to identify potential obstacles, such as cravings or lack of time for meal prep, and create a plan to overcome them. This may include strategies such as meal prepping on weekends, finding healthy substitutes for your favorite foods, or enlisting the support of a friend or family member.

Staying Motivated and Accountable

Staying motivated and accountable is essential for lasting success. It can be helpful to track your progress, whether through a journal or a mobile app, to stay accountable and motivated. You can also enlist the support of a friend or family member, or join a support group, to help you stay on track.

In the next chapter, we'll dive into creating a personalized meal plan that suits your dietary needs and preferences. We'll also provide tips for meal prep and dining out, so you can stay on track even when you're busy or on the go.

Chapter 3: Creating Your Personalized Meal Plan

Creating a personalized meal plan is essential for sustainable weight loss. In this chapter, we'll explore how to determine your daily calorie needs, how to choose the right macronutrient balance for your goals, and how to create a meal plan that suits your dietary needs and preferences.

Determining Your Daily Calorie Needs

Determining your daily calorie needs is the first step in creating a personalized meal plan. There are several online calculators that can help you estimate your daily calorie needs based on your age, gender, height, weight, and activity level. Once you have an estimate of your daily calorie needs, you can adjust your calorie intake based on your weight loss goals.

Choosing the Right Macronutrient Balance

Choosing the right macronutrient balance is also important for weight loss. The optimal macronutrient balance depends on your individual needs and goals. For example, a higher protein diet may be more beneficial for building muscle and promoting weight loss, while a higher carbohydrate diet may be more beneficial for athletes or individuals with high energy needs.

Creating a Meal Plan that Suits Your Needs and Preferences

Creating a meal plan that suits your needs and preferences is essential for sticking to your weight loss goals. You can start by creating a list of your favorite healthy foods, and incorporating them into your meal plan. It's also important to include a variety of foods from all food groups to ensure you're getting all the nutrients your body needs.

The Weight Loss Diet Plan

Losing weight is often a challenging process, but it doesn't have to be. One effective way to lose weight is by changing your diet. By making some simple dietary changes, you can reduce your calorie intake and start shedding those extra pounds. Here are some tips on how to go about it as a daily routine:

- **Count your calories**

The first step to losing weight is to understand how many calories you need to consume each day. This will depend on your gender, age, weight, height, and activity level. Once you know your daily calorie requirement, you can start tracking your calorie intake using a food diary or a calorie tracking app.

- **Choose nutrient-dense foods**

When trying to lose weight, it's important to choose foods that are high in nutrients and low in calories. Some examples of nutrient-dense foods include fruits, vegetables, whole grains, lean proteins, and low-fat dairy products. These foods will help you feel fuller for longer and provide your body with the nutrients it needs.

- **Reduce your portion sizes**

Portion control is crucial when trying to lose weight. Try using smaller plates, measuring your food, and avoiding eating straight out of the bag or container. This will help you avoid overeating and reduce your calorie intake.

- **Cut back on unhealthy fats and sugars**

High-fat and high-sugar foods are typically high in calories and low in nutrients. Avoid processed foods, fried foods, sugary drinks, and desserts as much as possible. Instead, opt for healthier fats like those found in nuts, seeds, and avocados, and natural sugars found in fruits.

- **Stay hydrated**

Drinking plenty of water throughout the day can help you feel fuller and reduce your calorie intake. Aim for at least eight glasses of water per day, and avoid sugary drinks and alcohol as much as possible.

- **Plan ahead**

Planning your meals and snacks in advance can help you make healthier choices and avoid compulsive eating. Make a grocery list, prep meals and snacks in advance, and pack healthy snacks to take with you when you're on the go.

By incorporating these dietary changes into your daily routine, you can lose weight and improve your overall health. Keep in mind that losing weight requires time and consistency.

Meal Prep and Dining Out Tips

Meal prep and dining out can be challenging when trying to lose weight. However, there are several strategies that can help you stay on track. For example, meal prepping on weekends can help ensure you have healthy meals ready to go during the week. When dining out, you can look for healthy options on the menu, ask for substitutions or modifications, and watch your portion sizes.

In the next chapter, we'll explore the importance of exercise for weight loss, and provide tips for creating a workout plan that suits your goals and fitness level.

Chapter 4: Making Healthy Choices Every Day

Making healthy choices every day is essential for sustainable weight loss. In this chapter, we'll explore how to make healthy choices when grocery shopping, cooking at home, and dining out. We'll also provide tips for staying motivated and avoiding common pitfalls.

Healthy Choices When Grocery Shopping
Making healthy choices when grocery shopping is key to sticking to your meal plan. Some tips for making healthy choices include sticking to the perimeter of the grocery store, choosing fresh fruits and vegetables, selecting lean protein sources, and avoiding processed foods and sugary drinks.

Healthy Choices When Cooking at Home

Cooking at home is a great way to control the ingredients and portions of your meals. Some tips for making healthy choices when cooking at home include using healthy cooking methods, such as grilling or baking, using herbs and spices for flavor instead of salt, and choosing healthy fats, such as olive oil or avocado oil.

Healthy Choices When Dining Out

Dining out can be challenging when trying to make healthy choices. However, there are a number of tactics that can be useful. Some tips for making healthy choices when dining out include choosing grilled or baked protein sources, asking for dressings and sauces on the side, and avoiding fried or creamy dishes.

The importance of Mindfulness and Self-awareness

Mindfulness and self-awareness are important for weight loss and overall health and well-being. Here's why:

- **Helps you identify triggers:** Mindfulness and self-awareness can help you identify triggers for unhealthy eating habits or behaviors. By being aware of your thoughts and emotions, you can recognize when you're tempted to overeat or make unhealthy choices and take steps to avoid those situations.

- **Encourages healthy decision-making:** When you're mindful and self-aware, you're more likely to make healthy decisions. You're able to recognize when you're hungry or full, and make choices that align with your goals and values.

- **Reduces stress**: Mindfulness and self-awareness can help reduce stress and promote relaxation. This can help prevent stress-related eating and improve overall health.

- **Improves body awareness**: Being mindful and self-aware can help you better connect with your body and its needs. This can help you tune into hunger and fullness cues, make informed choices about what to eat, and engage in physical activity that feels good for your body.

- **Encourages self-compassion:** Mindfulness and self-awareness can also encourage self-compassion. Instead of beating yourself up for mistakes or setbacks, you can approach challenges with kindness and understanding.

Incorporating mindfulness and self-awareness into your daily routine can help support your weight loss goals and improve your overall health and well-being. Simple practices like meditation, journaling, or breathing exercises can help you cultivate these important skills.

Strategies for Managing Cravings and Emotional Eating

Cravings and emotional eating can be major obstacles to weight loss and healthy eating habits. However, there are several strategies that can help you manage these challenges:

- **Identify your triggers:** Pay attention to the situations, emotions, or activities that trigger your cravings or emotional eating. This can help you recognize when you're vulnerable to these behaviors and prepare to manage them in a healthy way.

- **Find healthy alternatives:** Instead of giving in to unhealthy cravings or emotional eating, find healthy alternatives that satisfy your cravings or provide comfort. For example, if you're craving something sweet, try a piece of fruit or a small serving of dark chocolate.

- **Practice mindful eating:** Mindful eating entails being aware of your food, appreciating each mouthful, and consuming methodically. This can help you tune in to your body's hunger and fullness cues, and reduce the likelihood of overeating or emotional eating.

- **Control your stress:** Emotional eating has a lot of stress as a significant cause. Finding healthy ways to manage stress, such as exercise, meditation, or deep breathing, can help you avoid turning to food for comfort.

- **Get support:** Talking to a friend, family member, or therapist about your cravings and emotional eating can help you process your emotions and find healthier ways to cope.

Remember, managing cravings and emotional eating is a process that takes time and effort. Be patient with yourself, and don't be afraid to seek help or support when you need it. With consistent effort and healthy habits, you can overcome these challenges and achieve your weight loss goals.

Tips for keeping on course when life becomes hectic

Maintaining healthy habits can be challenging when life gets busy, but there are several tips that can help you stay on track:

- **Plan ahead:** Take some time each week to plan your meals, schedule your workouts, and prioritize your self-care. This can help you stay organized and focused, and reduce the likelihood of getting derailed by a busy schedule.

- **Keep healthy snacks on hand:** When you're short on time, it can be tempting to grab unhealthy snacks or fast food. Keep healthy snacks on hand, such as nuts, fruit, or pre-cut vegetables, to help you stay nourished and avoid unhealthy choices.

- **Make movement a priority:** Even if you can't make it to the gym or your regular workout class, find ways to incorporate movement into your day. Take a walk during your lunch break, do some stretching or yoga at home, or incorporate short bursts of activity throughout your day.

- **Get enough sleep:** Lack of sleep can disrupt your hormones and metabolism, making it harder to maintain healthy habits. Prioritize sleep by setting a consistent bedtime and creating a relaxing bedtime routine.

- **Simplify your meals:** Healthy eating doesn't have to be complicated or time-consuming. Focus on simple, nutritious

meals that can be prepared quickly, such
as salads, stir-fries, or roasted vegetables.

Remember, it's okay to be flexible and adjust
your routines when life gets busy. Don't beat
yourself up if you slip up or miss a workout –
just focus on getting back on track as soon as
you can. With consistent effort and healthy
habits, you can maintain your progress even
during busy times.
Staying motivated and avoiding common pitfalls
is essential for lasting success. Some tips for
staying motivated include setting short-term
goals, tracking your progress, and rewarding
yourself for reaching milestones. Common
pitfalls to avoid include emotional eating,
skipping meals, and falling into a rut with your
meal plan.

In the next chapter, we'll explore the importance
of exercise for weight loss, and provide tips for
creating a workout plan that suits your goals and
fitness level.

Chapter 5: Incorporating Exercise into Your Weight Loss Journey

Every weight reduction path needs to include exercise. In this chapter, we'll explore the benefits of exercise for weight loss, and provide tips for creating a workout plan that suits your goals and fitness level.

Benefits of Exercise for Weight Loss

Exercise provides a variety of benefits for weight loss. It helps to increase your metabolism, build lean muscle mass, and improve cardiovascular health. It can also improve your mood and reduce stress, which can help you stay motivated and on track with your weight loss goals.

Creating a Workout Plan

Creating a workout plan that suits your goals and fitness level is essential for success. Some factors to consider when creating a workout plan include your fitness level, schedule, and preferences. Some tips for creating a workout plan include starting with low-impact exercises and gradually increasing the intensity, incorporating strength training exercises, and finding activities that you enjoy.

Choosing the right types of exercise for your goals and preferences:

There are a variety of things to choose from when it comes to working out. To help you choose the right types of exercise for your goals and preferences, consider the following factors:

- **Goals**: Think about what you want to achieve through exercise. Do you want to build strength, improve cardiovascular health, or lose weight? Different types of exercise can be more effective for different goals.

- **Preferences:** Consider what types of activities you enjoy, as you're more likely to stick with an exercise routine that you find enjoyable. Do you prefer team sports, solo workouts, or outdoor activities?

- **Fitness level:** Be honest with yourself about your current fitness level, and choose activities that are appropriate for your level of fitness. Gradually increasing the intensity and duration of your workouts can help you avoid injury and build endurance.

- **Lifestyle:** Consider your lifestyle and schedule when choosing types of exercise. If you have limited time, high-intensity interval training (HIIT) or short, intense workouts may be more practical.

Some examples of different types of exercise and their benefits include:

Strength training: Builds muscle mass, improves bone density, and increases metabolism.
Cardiovascular exercise: Improves heart and lung health, burns calories, and can improve mood.
Yoga: Increases flexibility, improves balance, and can reduce stress.
Outdoor activities: Provides exposure to fresh air and nature, and can improve mental health and mood.
Remember, the most important thing is to choose types of exercise that you enjoy and that fit into your lifestyle. You can accomplish your exercise objectives and keep up a healthy, active lifestyle with perseverance and dedication.

Staying Motivated and Avoiding Common Pitfalls

Staying motivated and avoiding common pitfalls is essential for success. Some tips for staying motivated include setting realistic goals, tracking your progress, and finding a workout buddy or accountability partner. Common pitfalls to avoid include overtraining, not allowing for rest days, and not challenging yourself enough during workouts.

Strategies for staying active and motivated

- **Set realistic goals:** Establish achievable goals that are tailored to your fitness level and lifestyle. Start out simple and gradually increase the duration and difficulty of your workouts.

- **Find a workout buddy:** Working out with a friend can make exercise more enjoyable and keep you accountable.

- **Mix up your routine:** Variety can help prevent boredom and keep you motivated. Try new types of exercise or switch up your routine to challenge yourself.

- **Track your progress:** Keep a record of your workouts and progress to see how far you've come. This may inspire you and aid in your perseverance.

- **Celebrate your successes:** Celebrate your achievements and milestones, no matter how small. This can help you stay positive and motivated.

- **Make it a habit:** Incorporate exercise into your daily routine and make it a habit. Establish a regular exercise plan and follow it.

- **Reward yourself:** Set up rewards for reaching your fitness goals, such as treating yourself to a new workout outfit or a massage.

- **Focus on the benefits:** Remind yourself of the physical and mental health benefits

of exercise, such as improved mood,
energy, and overall health.

Remember, staying active and motivated is a journey, and it's okay to have setbacks or off days. The most important thing is to stay consistent and keep moving forward towards your goals. With dedication and perseverance, you can achieve a healthy, active lifestyle.

Incorporating Exercise into Your Daily Routine

Incorporating exercise into your daily routine can help you stay consistent with your workouts. Some tips for incorporating exercise into your daily routine include finding ways to be active throughout the day, such as taking the stairs instead of the elevator, and scheduling when it is most practical for you to perform your routines.

In the final chapter, we'll provide tips for maintaining your weight loss success and living a healthy, sustainable lifestyle.

Chapter 6: Navigating Challenges and Plateaus

Navigating challenges and plateaus is an important part of any weight loss journey. In this chapter, we'll explore common challenges and plateaus that can occur during the weight loss process, and provide tips for overcoming them.

Common Challenges During Weight Loss

There are several challenges that can occur during the weight loss process, such as emotional eating, lack of motivation, and social pressures. Some tips for overcoming these challenges include identifying triggers for emotional eating, finding ways to stay motivated, and communicating your goals and needs to your friends and family.

Common challenges that arise during weight loss:

- **Plateaus:** Weight loss plateaus can be frustrating and demotivating, but they're a natural part of the weight loss process. To overcome a plateau, try changing up your exercise routine or reducing your calorie intake.
- **Cravings and hunger:** Feeling hungry or experiencing food cravings is a common challenge during weight loss. To manage these challenges, try eating more filling foods, such as protein and fiber-rich foods, or schedule small, frequent meals throughout the day.
- **Emotional eating:** Emotional eating is using food to cope with stress or negative emotions. To overcome emotional eating, try identifying your triggers and finding alternative ways to cope with your emotions, such as exercise or meditation.
- **Social pressure:** Social pressure can make it difficult to stick to a healthy diet and exercise routine. To manage this challenge, try communicating your goals

and boundaries with friends and family, or find a supportive community to help you stay accountable.

- **Time constraints:** Busy schedules and competing priorities can make it difficult to find time for exercise and meal preparation. To overcome this challenge, try incorporating physical activity into your daily routine, or meal prepping on weekends to save time during the week.

Remember, weight loss is a journey with its ups and downs. It's important to stay patient and persistent, and to celebrate your successes along the way. By staying committed to your goals and addressing common challenges as they arise, you can achieve sustainable weight loss and a healthier lifestyle.

Dealing with Plateaus

Plateaus are a common occurrence during weight loss, and can be frustrating. Some tips for overcoming plateaus include increasing the intensity of your workouts, adjusting your calorie intake, and trying new types of exercises or activities.

Strategies for overcoming plateaus and setbacks during weight loss:

- **Reassess your goals**: If you've hit a plateau, it may be time to reassess your goals and adjust your plan accordingly. Consider setting new goals or revising your current plan to break through the plateau.

- **Switch up your routine:** To overcome a plateau, try changing up your exercise routine or trying a new type of exercise. This can help shock your body out of its routine and promote weight loss.

- **Adjust your calorie intake:** If you've hit a plateau, you may need to adjust your calorie intake. Try reducing your calorie intake slightly to promote weight loss.

- **Focus on non-scale victories:** Plateaus can be demotivating, but it's important to focus on non-scale victories, such as improved energy levels or increased endurance. These small wins can help you stay motivated and positive.

- **Manage stress:** Stress can contribute to weight loss plateaus and setbacks. To manage stress, try incorporating relaxation techniques, such as meditation or yoga, into your routine.

- **Get support:** Surround yourself with a supportive community, such as a weight loss support group, to help you stay accountable and motivated during plateaus and setbacks.

Remember, weight loss plateaus and setbacks are a normal part of the process. It's important to stay patient and persistent, and to continue working towards your goals. By trying new strategies, staying positive, and seeking support when needed, you can overcome plateaus and setbacks and achieve sustainable weight loss.

Maintaining Weight Loss Success

Maintaining weight loss success is essential for long-term health and wellness. Some tips for maintaining weight loss success include continuing to track your progress, setting new goals, and finding ways to stay motivated and engaged with your healthy lifestyle.

Living a Sustainable Lifestyle

Living a sustainable lifestyle is key to maintaining weight loss success. Some tips for living a sustainable lifestyle include finding healthy and enjoyable activities, making healthy food choices, and finding a balance between work, social life, and self-care.

Conclusion

Congratulations on completing **"The Ultimate Guide to Sustainable Weight Loss: A Comprehensive Diet Plan for Lasting Results"!** We hope this book has provided you with the knowledge, tools, and motivation you need to achieve your weight loss goals and maintain a healthy weight for life.

Celebrating Your Progress

Remember to celebrate your progress and successes along the way, no matter how small they may seem. Consistent effort and dedication to healthy habits will pay off in the long run, and you should be proud of yourself for taking this step towards a healthier, happier life.

Celebrating your progress and successes is an important part of the weight loss journey. It can help you stay motivated, boost your self-confidence, and reinforce healthy habits. Here are some ways to celebrate your progress and successes:

- **Treat yourself:** Treat yourself to something special when you reach a milestone or achieve a goal. This could be something as simple as a relaxing bath or a new piece of workout gear.

- **Share your success:** Share your success with friends and family or your support group. It can be encouraging to hear positive feedback from others and can help you stay motivated.

- **Take progress photos:** Taking progress photos can be a great way to see how far you've come and celebrate your progress.

- **Celebrate non-scale victories**: Celebrate non-scale victories, such as increased energy levels, improved sleep, or fitting into a smaller size clothing. These victories are just as important as the number on the scale.

- **Reflect on your journey**: Take time to reflect on your journey, the progress you've made, and the challenges you've overcome. This can help reinforce your commitment to your goals and inspire you to keep going.

Remember, weight loss is not just about reaching a number on the scale. Celebrating your progress and successes along the way is key to staying motivated and committed to your goals.

Maintaining A Healthy Weight For Life

Maintaining a healthy weight for life requires a commitment to a sustainable lifestyle that includes regular exercise, healthy food choices, and self-care. By continuing to track your progress, setting new goals, and staying motivated and engaged with your healthy lifestyle, you can achieve lasting success.

Maintaining a healthy weight for life requires making sustainable changes to your lifestyle. Here are some tactics that could be useful:

Continue to follow a healthy meal plan: Continue to follow a healthy meal plan that includes a variety of nutrient-dense foods and limits processed and high-calorie foods.

- **Keep moving:** Continue to incorporate physical activity into your daily routine. Find activities you enjoy and make them a regular part of your day.

- **Monitor your weight:** Regularly monitoring your weight can help you catch any potential changes and make adjustments as needed.

- **Manage stress:** Stress can lead to overeating and unhealthy habits. Incorporate stress-management techniques

into your daily routine, such as meditation
or yoga.

- **Get enough sleep:** Getting enough sleep
  is important for weight management.
  Strive for 7-8 hours of slumber per night,
  minimum.

- **Have a support system:** Continue to
  surround yourself with a supportive
  community, such as friends, family, or a
  weight loss support group.

- **Practice self-care:** Taking care of
  yourself is important for maintaining a
  healthy weight for life. Incorporate
  activities you enjoy, such as reading or
  hobbies, into your daily routine.

Remember, maintaining a healthy weight for life
is a journey, and it's important to continue to
prioritize your health and well-being even after
reaching your weight loss goals. By making
sustainable lifestyle changes and practicing self-

care, you can achieve long-term success and a healthier, happier life.

Thank you for choosing "The Ultimate Guide to Sustainable Weight Loss: A Comprehensive Diet Plan for Lasting Results" as your guide on this journey. We wish you all the best in your continued success and happiness!

Please help us leave a positive review so we can get to many people to eradicate unhealthy weight and disease associated with it from the world.